PREFACE

When I was 15 years old, my father and I took an airplane trip from Atlanta, Georgia to Hartford, Connecticut. We then proceeded to purchase an old red Buick from my Grandfather for pennies on the dollar. This was followed by a thirteen hour drive back to Atlanta. What intrigued me about the trip, was that my father slept pretty much the whole way. Occasionally, I would look over and see him smiling with that "I just got a great deal" look on his face. He was very trusting, given the fact I had only had my learners permit for approximately three days. I felt like king of the road driving down the East Coast and it gave me an incredible sense of independence.

Occasionally, he would wake up and give me words of wisdom about driving and life in general. During one of these periods of consciousness, my father said something to me that I never forgot. He told me to concentrate on myself, educate myself, and treat others well. He told me there would come a time in life that would be my "Eureka!" moment. He described this as a moment in time when I would discover a great truth that only hard work and education would provide.

My "Eureka!" moment came approximately 14 years later when I was doing my chief residency in Orthopedic Surgery at the Georgia Baptist Medical Center. This book is about that moment. I've waited 19 years to write the book because I needed to make sure that what I was thinking, was backed up by science. I've chosen this moment in time to write this book and share with you one of the most extraordinary aspects of medicine that I have ever seen over the years. I hope the information I share with you will lead you to a better understanding of the future of medicine. In this book I use the word Stems to represent stem cells and the products they create in our bodies.

I dedicate this book to my father, Rudolph Price, who has long since passed but lives on in my daily thoughts.

CHAPTER 1: THE INITIATION

In 1992, I left the sheltered world of medical school in Augusta, Georgia to embark on a brutal initiation into the world of medicine.

On July 1,1992, I showed up at the Georgia Baptist Medical Center in Atlanta ready to start my surgical internship, which was one year long. I was feeling pretty good with my new white jacket, stethoscope, and reflex hammer. I thought I would just be able to walk around the halls of the hospital and people would do whatever I said, and patients would have the utmost of respect for me. At about seven thirty in the morning on my first day of work I quickly realized that this concept had been raked over the coals and died a lonely death. By eight thirty I was holding retractors for a vascular surgeon using all my strength for three hours while staring at the ceiling. I started to wonder if I'd made the correct decision about medical school and surgical residency. I was even further convinced that I had made the wrong decision when at about 10 o'clock that night I was still in the Operating Room being yelled at, bled on, and subsequently vomited on by a patient in the recovery room. By the time I got home that night, my entire four years of medical school seemed like a dream world with expectations that would never be met.

The second day of my internship was not much different. In fact, it began at five thirty in the morning by visiting the surgical patients I had assisted with the day before. I didn't recognize the patients of course because when I had seen them last I didn't see their faces but rather deep into their belly while surgical procedures were being performed. It was during the second day that I got to see patient's faces and talk with them that I decided to stick it out. The patients were very grateful, humble, and thankful. This was despite the fact that their abdomens had been opened up and exposed to an entire room while a surgeon barked orders and proceeded to remove parts of their body the day before. The previous day became more acceptable knowing there had been good surgical results. It was by the end of the second day of my internship that I was completely invested in the concept of spending the next five years of my life being yelled at, sleep deprived, and tireless hours spent within the confines of a hospital.

As the months went by, my lifestyle adjusted to work, sleep, and occasional exercise. There really was nothing more to life than that for quite a while. Those around me suffered the same fate with no exposure to the sun. By Christmas, everyone around me looked pale, scrawny, and had lost their girlfriends or were going through a divorce. Many times I wondered if this was a reasonable way to treat a human being, but then again, a certain twisted corner of my mind enjoyed the abuse.

Being in a surgical internship essentially means that you are the bottom of the totem pole. Anyone in the hospital with a badge can yell at you and you can't say a word back. When I say badge, I mean the cleaning crew, the physicians, and the nurses in the operating room. I remember watching Full Metal Jacket and feeling like I now understood what the first six weeks of boot camp was like in the military.

In the spring of my first year of my surgical internship, I did a rotation in Orthopedic Surgery, which would soon be my chosen profession. I'm not quite sure how it happened but I managed to even be yelled at by the parking lot attendant on this crisp spring morning. While I walked into the hospital with my head down shoulders slouched, I looked up to see the first smiling face I had seen in almost 9 months. It was one of the senior attending surgeons, John Keating MD. He actually shook my hand and invited me to breakfast. I thought perhaps I was about to be fired or asked to do some monumentally degrading task and this was my last supper prior to that request. As it turned out, Dr. Keating was very pleasant and actually spoke with me as if I were a human being. He talked about martial arts as well as some of the more literary works in our American culture. I found the conversation exhilarating given the fact that #1 I wasn't being yelled at, and #2 I was actually being treated as a colleague.

After our conversations about world matters and political issues of the day, he turned my attention back to medicine. When he spoke with me, he talked about a procedure that he had started performing that no one would accept anytime soon, and that he would take a lot of criticism for performing. He told me about the procedure called a sacroiliac fixation/fusion. He told me that in America the common concept in people with back pain was that they had a disc herniation and that they needed surgery. He went on to explain to me that in his opinion, a lot of spine surgery was performed that was inappropriate and in fact, bordered on criminal activity. Dr. Keating explained to me how a great number of patients with low back pain, actually had problems with their sacroiliac joint which is the joint on either side of the low back, in the area behind the hip. Although I had been through medical school and learned about the sacroiliac joint, I had never once heard anyone say that the sacroiliac joint was a source of low back pain. I started to wonder if I was speaking to someone that was perhaps merely pontificating about ideas he had regarding low back pain but that he would never actually perform the procedure to treat the sacroiliac joint.

A couple weeks later when we were given our surgical assignments of the morning I was surprised to learn I had been assigned to Dr. Keating and his surgical room for the day. Our first case that morning was a sacroiliac joint fixation procedure. We proceeded to place the patient on their stomach and prepare the low back and hip region for a surgical procedure. I usually would have read up and studied on what type of surgery we would do that day, but in this case nothing existed for me to read or study.

The surgical procedure took about 30 minutes and only required two small incisions about the length of a pencil tip. He then proceeded to drill across the pelvic bone and into the spinal column. Under X-ray he then placed two screws across the joint. As we completed the procedure I looked up with a little bit of bewilderment as to what we had just done and what result should we expect. Given the fact that we had merely placed two screws across a large joint so quickly I had my doubts.

Approximately 30 minutes after the surgery was complete I visited the patient in the recovery room to do my routine orders. I was shocked when the patient actually stood up and walked across the floor to use the restroom on her own. I looked around the room to see if the nurses were about to yell at me for allowing the patient to walk. One of the more friendly nurses saw my anxiety and reassured me that "this is how Dr. Keating's patients normally respond to surgery." I then became very intrigued with the entire procedure and ended up spending the next four years doing clinical research with Dr. Keating as well as following patients with him in the office who had low back pain. During those four years I noticed Dr. Keating was often not invited to some of the more established orthopedic surgeon's meetings and the other doctors did not socialize with him much. In fact, some of the other surgeons would often make off hand comments about Dr. Keating operating on the lunatic fringe and performing unfounded surgical procedures. To the contrary I knew that whatever Dr. Keating was doing was working so well that the patients were up walking almost immediately after surgery. This included patients that were having to use crutches or a cane leading up to the surgery.

As I became more aware of what was going on during the surgical procedure that we were performing, I started to wonder if it was the screws that were being placed across the joint or the drilling of the joint that was actually making the patient feel better. I now know that it was both that made the patients feel better. The reality is while drilling across the joint, stems (stem cells) from the pelvis were being leaked into the sacroiliac joint. As the screws were being placed through the drill holes it carried even more stems into the joint. It took me another 15 years to realize it, but in fact the stems that had leaked into the joint were almost certainly the main reason the patients felt almost immediate relief in the recovery room. Certainly the screws helped stabilize the sacroiliac joint and pelvis but two screws alone did not mechanically have the ability to provide enough stability to give the type of pain relief that I witnessed in these patients.

As I proceeded through residency I couldn't help but notice that anytime I was fixing a bone by drilling into the bone and placing screws, plates, or other various forms of hardware, that there was always a leaking of bone marrow contents into the wound and fracture site. The contents of the bone marrow would not only leak into and around the bone but into the tissues surrounding the bone, which included muscles, ligaments and tendons. I then started wondering why when we performed X-rays within the weeks following surgery the bone would heal, but the tissues that the bone marrow leaked into would not develop areas of bone. When some of those patients were brought back for follow up procedures in subsequent years and a repeat incision was made to remove screws and plates I was startled to find that there was no bone formation in the muscles, ligaments, and tendons. I then started wondering how bone marrow could leak into the areas within a fractured bone and it would turn into bone, but this same bone marrow would leak into tendons, ligaments and muscle and NOT form bone. This question plagued me for many years.

As the years in residency wore on, and I rose through the ranks , I eventually had my choice as to which attending surgeons I would assist and which surgeons I would assign to the lower level residents for the day. I found myself electively choosing to work with doctor Keating and his sacroiliac joint work as well as his other surgical procedures. I'd always felt a loyalty to him given the fact that he was pleasant to me when no one else was and he had allowed me to assist him in his surgical procedures as a colleague. By the time I had reached my chief residency year, Dr. Keating's procedure had become more popular and his office was extremely busy with patients who had undergone low back surgeries that did not work and he would then perform sacroiliac joint procedures on many of these patients and much to the delight of the patient there would be good relief and sometimes near full pain relief by performing the sacroiliac surgery. It was quite clear to me that there was something going on behind the scenes with bone marrow that had some special place in medicine.

CHAPTER 2: FAMILY HISTORY

My Grandmother's name was Rose, but don't let the name fool you. She would just as soon punch you in the nose as hold a conversation with you if you threatened her family. She was very loyal to her family and very loving to my sister and I. We would travel from Atlanta to Philadelphia, sometimes up to 3 times a year, to visit with her and my Grandfather in their Polish neighborhood on the east side of Philadelphia.

The diet of the Polish neighborhood generally consisted of either pizza or salami sandwiches followed by large pieces of cake or pie. Once you had washed it all down with a carbonated beverage it was time to pull out a pack of cigarettes and work your way half through the pack while talking away the evening until passing out. This lifestyle was very perplexing to me and I soon came to wonder if any vegetables were served in Philadelphia.

At my home in Atlanta it was extremely unusual to see any sign of pizza or salami and I wondered if this was some kind of geographical anomaly. I soon came to realize that this was actually the choice of my grandparents to eat these comfort foods that immigrants enjoyed as a happy ending to long arduous days. Unfortunately, these foods did nothing to build up the immune system or keep the bone marrow and Stems healthy.

For a while I thought that this diet was probably just as good as any other given the fact that my Grandmother was strong and when we went to Philadelphia Flyers hockey games she would often yell and strong arm the fiercest of males sitting nearby if they dared cheer for the other team. When we walked down the street, she walked a straight line and anyone in her way found themselves veering in another direction as to not encounter her wrath or impede her progress to her final destination.

As the years wore on and I started visiting her more in her older age, I recognized that she started having signs of multiple medical problems including diabetes, high blood pressure, stroke, and unfortunately, major heart diseases. It was quite clear that the diet had a lot to do with these medical problems, however it didn't dawn on me at the time that the reason for these medical conditions had a lot to do with inflammation of not only liver and kidneys but also of the lining of the blood vessels. As I progressed in school during my medical training I recognized that the inflammation of blood vessels and heart had certainly lead to the multiple medical conditions which my grandmother experienced which included her ultimate demise from cardiac failure. It was only her strong genetic predisposition, will to survive, and provide for her family that kept her going as long as it did but I cant help but think that she would've lasted longer and would've been healthier in her final years if a simple few rules had been followed. These days with the availability of information at our fingertips, most people are well aware of what they should or shouldn't consume. Most of us have been well educated on why certain foods aren't good and why others promote health. In fact, there are many foods that are actual anti-inflammatory foods and this includes such foods as blueberries, broccoli, yogurt, and even water. Adhering to the basic principle of eating anti-inflammatory foods, and avoiding those foods that cause inflammation has been shown without question to prolong life and decrease disease.

Stems, as we are now aware, have a significant anti-inflammatory effect and exert that effect in our bodies on a daily basis. Take for example the simple act of falling down and scraping your knee. That wound will stop bleeding within a few minutes as the platelets in your body rush to that site to clot the wound, creating a scab. These cells bring in inflammatory factors that increase swelling and pain at that site as the tissues begin to fight infection and halt the loss of blood. One of the final stages in wound healing is that the initial cells that came to the site causing the inflammation then send out a signal to the

Stems in our bodies. The Stems that already exist in our bodies respond by making their way to the site of the injury and initiate an anti-inflammatory effect during the process of healing the tissues. The simple truth is there is no machine that has ever been made that can match the efficiency and healing properties of our own bodies when they're in good health.

As I have mentioned with regard to foods, it is absolutely essential that every individual be aware of which foods cause inflammation. The very food that's placed in your body each day can alter and shape your future far more than you ever imagined.

We can all agree that it would be wonderful to look and feel great for as long in life as possible. The problem is, the daily grind of adhering to diets and lifestyle that keep us healthy are difficult to maintain.

If we have more knowledge about the inflammatory effects of the foods they eat I believe a drastic change in eating habits would occur. I give you the example of my grandmother. The fact is, she just did not have the knowledge about why the foods she was eating were not good for her, and why the smoking and excessive drinking lead to poor health. I'm sure she had been given a hard time about it many times but until the knowledge is there the fear doesn't exist.

For example, if you were told that when you woke up every morning and ate a bowl of red chili that you would be healthy, live longer, and feel better, whereas, if you ate a bowl of green chili you would feel bad all day and live a short life, the choice would be very clear. The problem with food and healthy lifestyle choices is there is a lot of gray area. If we will recognize the exact foods that increase inflammation in our body versus the foods that decrease inflammation in our body we will have a better understanding and knowledge of which food is good and why. This also applies to exercise, sleep, and any aspect of social life, including emotions and interpersonal relationships.

If you think about it, from the moment you wake up in the morning until the moment you go to bed at night you are either being inflamed by some situation, or you are calm and relaxed. There really is no in-between. The objective would be to wake up in the morning and begin the day with anti-inflammatory foods, have anti-inflammatory relationships, and be surrounded with calm work conditions. Certainly this is an idealistic view and I have not met anyone that has been able to exist in this anti-inflammatory state all day long. However, having the knowledge of how these inflamed social situations along with diet, and sleep patterns effect us gives us more knowledge and discipline regarding what will keep us healthier longer. Going back to my Grandmother in Philadelphia, I recognized that her days were stressful from the moment she woke up until she came home from work. Even when she got home from work, due to the fact that she didn't make much money the stress really did not stop. Constant concerns about finances, supporting the family, and providing for the children created an inflammatory psychological environment for my grandparents. I eventually became convinced that the unhealthy diets that my grandparents and their neighbors enjoyed on a nightly basis were nothing more than comfort foods. Those comfort foods gave an instant feeling of a high, or sugar rush, followed by a long nights sleep only to get up and do it all again. The food, smoking, and drinking was nothing more than a psychological and physical crutch to get some sort of feeling of relaxation or comfort, even if only for a moment. Unfortunately what my grandparents and most people don't recognize is that these comfort foods and drinks are nothing more than inflammatory producing agents in the body. They have long-term effects that include inflammation of the liver, kidneys, stomach, and linings of the arteries and veins.

It was uncanny how much cardiac and pulmonary disease existed in that Polish immigrant neighborhood in Philadelphia. If only they had the knowledge that healthy anti-inflammatory diets would have helped them cope with life and adversity in a much better way and provided for a longer healthier existence, I am confident that my Grandparents would have chosen that healthy lifestyle.

Commonly, diet and exercise follows a herd mentality. Take for example that Polish neighborhood in Philadelphia. If one person in that neighborhood chose to become healthy by eating well, sleeping well, stopping smoking and limiting their alcohol intake, most likely they would be the object of ridicule and be excluded from social activities in that neighborhood. Therefore, the herd mentality of "everyone's doing it, so I might as well so I can fit in" certainly applied just as much then as it does now. This peer pressure is a much stronger force than any of us could imagine. It guides our social interactions, diet, exercise and relationships. It is imperative that we learn to educate ourselves about inflammatory foods, relationships, and sleep patterns so that we can rise above the metabolic ups and downs that occur in our daily lives. You will be a much stronger individual if you learn this now and carry it through life.

CHAPTER 3: LONGEVITY

Greenville, Mississippi is a lonely, out of the way town sitting on the Mississippi river halfway between Vicksburg and Memphis. The people are friendly, and the cuisine is out of this world. It is miles from any major highway and seems to be a step back into the past.

In 2007 I had taken a job in Greenville for a two-year stint following my assignment as an Assistant Professor of Orthopedic Surgery at Emory University in Atlanta. The town, much to my surprise, was full of 90 plus year old people who still worked in the yard everyday, hunted, and could still cook up a storm. The first night I was at my house in Greenville there were no less than four knocks at the door with people presenting me with cakes, hot meals and deserts to give me a warm welcome to the community.

The first morning I was driving in Greenville, I was sitting at a red light and heard a loud screeching sound pull up in the lane beside me. Much to my surprise there was a gentleman dressed for a day at work, sitting on a riding lawnmower, using it as his primary form of transportation. As the day progressed and I was driving around town doing all the preparations for my new job, I was passed by more people riding lawnmowers. I was shocked that these individuals had rigged the riding lawnmowers to go up to speeds of 40mph. It was quite clear that I had arrived in one of the poorest county's in the United States and in some ways a step back in time.

The two years I spent in Greenville was an extraordinary immersion into the culture of the deep South, complete with hospitality, respect, and a gratifying feeling that I was actually doing some good when I showed up at the hospital at 2am for an emergency. Most injuries that patients experienced were from bar fights or slamming into each other on the highways.

The one thing that became very obvious while working in Greenville was it seemed like every other person I met was at least 70 years old and there were many people in their 90s that still remained very active. I would have a chance to occasionally sit down with these individuals as they came into the hospital for routine care, and I would ask them why it was that they were still working and remaining socially active at such an advanced age. Overwhelmingly the response was that the moment you stop taking care of your health you start to die. It was almost as if there was a private sect of people in Greenville who understood the secret to long life. I compared this to other areas where I had worked and lived where the average income was double or triple that of Greenville and it became clear to me that one does not have to be wealthy to live a healthy lifestyle. Occasionally, one of these elderly individuals would fall or be in a motor vehicle accident and have a pelvis or hip fracture. Many times I would have to take these individuals to the operating room to perform repairs or replacements of joints. I couldn't help but notice that in these very active, elderly individuals, their bone was just as hard as a patient in their forties. The marrow of the bone was very rich in blood supply and accepted screws and plates (hardware) very well without loosening. I thought perhaps something was in the water in Greenville that was responsible for this phenomenon. As it turns out, these were individuals that had lived in a community where the social norm was to remain active athletically, socially, and with employment for as long in life as they were able. It became evident to me that this was the source of their long life and more importantly, their healthy bones. As we now know in the field of medicine, healthy bones with dense marrow also equates to a high volume of stems. Stems as we are also aware, are the very cornerstone of anti-inflammatory agents in our bodies as well as healing factors that repair not only the outside wounds that we experience such as scrapes and cuts but also internal wounds that we experience on a day to day basis. The evidence that exists in the rheumatology and orthopedic literature that has become increasing more recognized is the ability of Stems to prevent cancers, diseases, and inflammation in our bodies.

Perhaps the individuals in Greenville, Mississippi can teach the rest of the world a lesson that old age is no excuse for retirement, but rather a reason to continue with a healthy lifestyle of exercise, employment, and an anti-inflammatory diet. I also found these elderly individuals to be very socially active in the local arts and school activities of their grandchildren and great grandchildren. The close families that these elderly individuals were a part of, in my opinion, were essential to helping maintain the social stimulation and structure that aided in the prolonged life that these individuals experienced.

Does an unhealthy lifestyle lead to aging, or does aging lead to an unhealthy lifestyle? Many people will rely on the fact that they are aging as an excuse for their poor health. The stark reality is that an unhealthy lifestyle leads to physiological aging. This is undeniable. Certainly it requires more discipline to maintain a healthy lifestyle and resist the ever-present temptation to use aging as an excuse.

The simple truth is that a healthy lifestyle including a balanced diet, social interactions, employment, and exercise, keep our bodies healthy by keeping the bones dense with a rich source of Stems. These Stems provide anti-inflammatory effects for the body and the ongoing ability to heal the wounds that our body suffers every day.

Very rarely does a day go by that I don't think about the individuals in Greenville, Mississippi who taught me to refuse to allow myself to age physiologically or accept any excuse for poor health. In the face of uncontrollable circumstances such as cancer and trauma, the body will fight better and live longer if it is physiologically young, and supported by a healthy supply of Stems.

CHAPTER 4: THE SMOKING GUN

I hate to admit it but when I was a teenager, I actually walked around with a pack of cigarettes rolled up in my white t-shirt sleeve. I remember vividly thinking that it would be a good way to attract the opposite sex. Unbelievably, it actually worked. This was the social thinking of the day consistent with Hollywood films, billboards, and magazine ads on every corner. The accepted treatment of many colds and other illness was a pack of cigarettes and cup of coffee.

I remember my grandparents, aunts, and uncles alike, having their morning breakfast consist of several cigarettes, a piece of toast with butter, and a cup of coffee. It wasn't until many years later that a group of Mississippi trial lawyers started garnering support from 40 attorney generals from other states as well as key members of the US Senate to lower the boom on the tobacco industry and expose the rampant lies being told.

I'm sure we can all remember flying across the country on a commercial flight with a smoking section and a non-smoking section separated by an invisible wall between two seats. Even though I accepted smoking as a form of diet and medical treatment it didn't change the fact that when someone blew smoke all over my clothes and hair something just didn't seem right. Even as a young kid flying amongst this smoke-filled air I suspected that I was being fooled and somehow this smoke was not good for my health. It wasn't long ago, that there were tennis tournaments sponsored by major tobacco companies such as Virginia Slims. I remember very well during my medical school years a movement that began to remove cigarette smoking advertising from sporting events. It didn't take long for this to happen after the movement began, but what was shocking was how long it took for someone to protest and litigate against the massive fraud that was propagated to our country by the cigarette companies.

We now know that there can be no more detrimental activity to our health than smoking and the use of tobacco products. The reality is that cigarette smoke, nicotine and everything associated with it destroys our immune system, bones and ultimately has a devastating effect on the Stems in our body. As I pointed out, Stems are the very key to keeping down inflammation and finishing off the healing process in our bodies for both internal and external wounds. Stems are so vital to healthy living that without them death would be imminent. I hate to be morbid but it is a fact that without the existence of Stems in our body we would quickly succumb to disease and inflammatory processes that would ultimately lead to our demise. It is scary to consider how much damage cigarettes and tobacco products have done to our society in the last 50 years.

What we should consider is that advertising to both adults and children for fast food is nearly as damaging to our health as the formerly accepted advertising of tobacco products. The fact that fast food chains and restaurants can submit commercials both on Saturday mornings in between cartoons, on cereal boxes, and billboards, appears to have the same fraudulent nature as those former tobacco efforts. If our society were somehow able to eliminate these fast food advertisements and chains then it is my firm belief that the health of our children would take a large leap forward. Think about the other children that go to school with your kids. Consider who the more intelligent and motivated kids are and you'll find that these are the kids with disciplined lifestyles with respect not only to diet, but homework, exercise, and consistent sleep patterns to support a long, healthy life. These patterns are established early on in childhood and are difficult to break. Similarly, bad habits that begin early in life are almost insurmountable as we grow up and tend to revert to some of the habits of our childhood that remind us of happier times. Particularly during times of stress, anxiety, and depression we crave the foods we ate during our carefree younger years.

You see, it's really a mentality that must take place and exist early on in life to set the course for a healthy lifespan. I'm always surprised how people ignore statistics and refer to the one 80 year-old person they know who smoked, drank, and ate fast food their entire life. My argument to that would be that if that same individual had led a healthy lifestyle they would've lived to see the age of 100. It's just a matter of genetics taking some people so far as to give false hope to those of us not blessed with world-class genetics. Rather it is better to concentrate on the more mundane statistical analysis that eating a poor diet and maintaining an unhealthy lifestyle leads to poor health, poor nutrition, and stems that just can't get the job done.

One phenomenon that we have in our country is multiple media outlets that are constantly looking for something to catch their reader or viewers attention. One prime example is the hot dog eating contest that takes place on national tv and makes heroes out of individuals who can consume 50 hotdogs in one sitting. The mentality that this produces in us as a society is that "hey this guy can eat 50 hotdogs, so I can eat 2 or 3 and be just fine." Once again statistics are being used against us. These are individuals who have a genetic ability to consume mass amounts of foods during that short period of time. That they can do so and maintain reasonable health is broadcast to us to influence further hotdog eating by the masses. What we are statistically unaware of is the fact that the average individual can't eat more than a few hotdogs, and if they did so everyday for a few years the health implications would be devastating.

Going back to the Mississippi trial attorneys who took on the tobacco industry money was clearly a motivating factor. The attorneys who garnered the support of attorney generals from around the country along with key members of the US senate made a full on assault on the tobacco industry, securing billions of dollars in settlements. It is so ingrained in our society to continue with unhealthy fast food diets that it would take not just a few attorneys, but rather legislation from the top to put a stop to the epidemic. It has been encouraging that some legislation has been passed in New York to decrease the visibility of large soft drinks to the unsuspecting public. I'm hoping that this is just the beginning.

A re-education of America is certainly in order. Everyone has heard that we have to stay away from unhealthy foods and stick to certain food groups to maintain health but it is my opinion that if America were further educated on what was actually happening inside our bodies the behavior patterns would change much quicker than not.

During my first year in medical school I was assigned was a cadaver. The cadaver was a local individual who dedicated their body for others to learn the practice of medicine. It was a great honor and privilege to be able to learn about the human body from the great gift that this individual provided. I remember comparing the livers, kidneys, and lungs of one cadaver to another. We were able to learn a little bit about the history of the individuals with regard to their health records and without exception those who smoked had lungs that looked like a black leathery handbag. It was quite evident those individuals who had not smoked as the lungs looked healthy, pink and had good blood supply. There were many times while I was performing the dissections when I wondered how certain individuals had even lived as long as they had given the fact that their lungs looked so shriveled. Certainly these individuals were not enjoying good health in their final years and most likely had chronic coughs, infections, lack of energy, decreased sex drive, and the inability to participate in a healthy lifestyle. The other thing

I often wondered when I was in the anatomy lab was what kind of example these individuals had given to not only their children but grandchildren as well. Were they propagating the unhealthy lifestyles that had led to their ultimate demise? Are we doomed to have more generations who consider this the accepted status quo of health? Money is a motivating factor for us not only for the basic needs that it supports but also the recreational activities that it affords. I like to compare Stems to money. There is an age-old phrase that I hear frequently from money managers which is "every dollar you have should be viewed as an employee that goes to work for you." You want to have your Stems work for you in the best way possible to maintain health. Smoking, poor diet, poor sleep habits, lack of social interactions, and unemployment does nothing but debilitate our Stems and decrease the ability to heal the wounds that occur on a daily basis. I believe that if we cared as much about the health of our Stems as we do our financial health, we would have a much different perspective on how we should conduct our lifestyles each day.

I invite you to join me in changing not only your own approach to daily living, but also to influence others to think about their own health by directing their attention to maintaining the health of their Stems. Healthy Stems have the ability to increase not only happiness and health, but also prolong an enjoyable active life.

CHAPTER 5: HOW WE MOVE

In order to have a good understanding about the type of treatments that help us, including Stems, it is important to understand how our joints move and function.

One thing that's important to remember is that most of our joints are layered with cartilage that has very poor blood supply. The blood supply gets less and less the closer it gets to the joint lining itself. A great deal of the nutrition that our cartilage receives is from the joint fluid, thus, the importance of maintaining healthy joints and joint fluid so our cartilage can remain healthy. In summary, cartilage relies on maintaining health by a direct blood supply and the joint fluid bathing the joint.

With regard to the shoulder, this is one of the most extraordinary mobile joints in our body. It moves in many directions and if the muscles surrounding the shoulder were not in good condition, the shoulder would fall out of joint under its own weight. The simple fact is there are ligaments and cartilage that make up the shoulder, but they are not strong enough to maintain its health, motion, and stability in our everyday activities. I am always surprised when I go to a gym to work out and see many individuals doing bench pressing and pushups and all other forms of power strengthening for the front portion of the shoulder and chest. It is surprising seeing that these same individuals don't spend the time strengthening the back of their shoulders, leading to poor balance and muscle control of the shoulder. The muscle imbalance that most individuals have of the shoulder contributes to abnormal sliding and motion of the joint which only advances conditions such as arthritis and bursitis (inflammation of the gel sack about the shoulder). Certainly power lifting, bench pressing, push ups, and fly exercises allow the individual to develop the muscles they can see in the mirror, but the difficulty is convincing someone to try and develop the muscles they cannot see in the mirror. Therefore, shoulder health relies on keeping all the muscles strengthened in both the front and back. Proper strengthening of the muscles in the front and back of the shoulder will indirectly keep the muscles in the top and bottom of the shoulder healthy as well. Adhering to this simple principal when going to the gym will contribute to a much healthier shoulder that moves with a much more normal motion leading to less inflammation down the road.

The elbow is a joint that seemingly moves in only 2 directions. The reality is the elbow also supports rotation of the forearm inward and outward (called pronation and supination). The most important thing to remember about the elbow is that since it does have some limitations to motion and is not as mobile as the shoulder it should be placed in a position of comfort when performing any exercises. Similar to the shoulder is the fact that the muscles on both the front and back of the elbow should be exercised in order to maintain proper health of the joint. Once again, it's easy to go to the gym and develop muscles you can see in the mirror, while it's harder to develop muscles you can't see in the mirror.

With regard to the wrist and hand the activities of developing wrist strength should be concentrated on more static activities. In other words to get a 20 pound weight and work on wrist flexion and extension to strengthen the forearm musculature is simply just not smart. The incredible stress that gets put on the wrist and the base of the thumb in performing wrist flexion and extension exercises against resistance, is a force that the wrist can only tolerate for so long before it starts to break down in a big way. For example, injuries to the cartilage, early arthritis, and degeneration of the wrist joint are common in gym enthusiasts.

With regard to the hips there is one crucial key to maintaining hip health. The range of motion must be maintained in the hips. It does the hip no good to do squats, hamstring curls, and other quad exercises if one is not maintaining range of motion of the hip. If you'll recall, we discussed how important joint fluid is to the nutrition of the joint. The less a joint goes through its full range of motion the less joint fluid is moved around the joint, and thus a less healthy joint is the result. In other words, I would rather see someone spend 20 minutes stretching out their hips and maintaining hip flexibility through gentle stretching exercises than hammering the hips with squats, leg presses, and other forms of significant stress on the hip without concentrating on maintaining range of motion.

The knee is perhaps the most injured and damaged joint in all of sports and everyday living activities. The knee is extremely vulnerable since the foot is usually planted on the ground and a tremendous amount of body weight stresses the knee in several directions despite the fact that the knee does not move naturally in these directions. The knee essentially moves from flexion into extension with some minimal amount of rotation that takes place. Think of the knee as a nutcracker. As the forces from the ground work from the foot side of the knee and the forces from your body weight work from the other side of the knee, it easy to see how the knee is easily injured with any abnormal twisting. The stability of the knee is primarily maintained by four ligaments. These four ligaments prevent abnormal motion to the front, back and sides of the knee. In a healthy individual these ligaments are very strong and can resist a lot of force but when the force of the upper body and the force of the ground exerts stress on the knee, much like a nutcracker, it is simply too much force for the knee to withstand.

The health of the knee is critical in maintaining normal lifestyle and participation in most job activities. The fact is, even a sitting position can put a tremendous amount of stress on the knee. The knee cap (patella) is pressed with a massive amount of force into the femur in a sitting position. This is the reason why many people get knee pain while sitting in a movie theater, their office, or at home. When you realize that the quadricep muscle is pulling the kneecap into the femur under a tremendous amount of force in the sitting position its easy to see how any injury to the cartilage under the kneecap can be extremely painful in the sitting position. In fact, individuals who have injuries to the cartilage underneath the kneecap would rather stand up and walk around than sit down for a long period of time. These cartilage injuries to the knee have been extremely difficult to remedy, despite some of the most advanced scientific minds in the world working to find solutions. There have been specific knee replacement procedures designed for this particular problem, but thus far there is no reliable, predictable treatment that will make an individual pain free or replace the original cartilage that was damaged with these injuries.

With regard to the ankle and foot it is easy to understand how the ankle gets injured if you apply the same principles for the knee that we discussed. When the ground is applying a force to the foot, the body weight can easily overwhelm the ankle with any abnormal motion. If you look down at your own ankle you will see that you can rotate your foot in a circular motion. This circular motion comes from not just one joint but the action of two joints. There's the ankle joint itself, and then there is another joint just below the ankle called the subtalar joint. When these two joints are healthy we find ourselves able to run straight, backwards, cut from one side to the other and tolerate significant forces in the ankle.

With regard to motion of the spine, the spine has essentially three joints at many levels from the neck down to the tailbone. These joints are also lined with cartilage and connective tissue that provide padding and gliding motions. The health and well being of the muscle around the spine has a great deal to do with keeping the discs healthy between each level in the spine as well as the cartilage. Most of us are already aware of significant injuries that can occur in the spine, which includes excessive lifting, not only with a single event, but also repetitive use over time.

With regard to all of these joints there is one simple common denominator. These joints rely heavily on maintaining motion and reducing stress in order to maintain healthy cartilage. As advanced as our society is in treating injuries and repairing damage no one has yet figured out how to grow cartilage in the human body. Certainly there have been some certain successes in the laboratory, but being able to do this in a live human body does not exist to any reliable degree.

As our cartilage is damaged and wears out either through aging or injury it gets thin and starts to expose the underlying bone. The body then tries to fight this damage with inflammation which is the first step in repair. The body does not know that it can't heal and regrow the cartilage but the inflammatory process initiates the attempt anyway. It is this inflammation that gives us the pain that we feel in damaged or injured joints. Most of us who have joint pain are familiar with the fact that sometimes we have a "good day" and sometimes we have a "bad day". Its easy to wonder why when a joint is damaged it can feel fine one day and the next day it can't even be moved. The simple explanation comes with the rhythmic inflammatory process of our body. For example, if you have an injured knee, the body attempts to repair the injured knee by initiating an inflammatory process. This process begins with certain proteins and enzymes reaching the knee through our bloodstream that initiate the repair process. Our body does not know that it cannot repair the cartilage but it attempts to do so anyway and sometimes can even leave some scar tissue in its place but can't recreate the original cartilage. The body goes through cyclical actions to try and heal the joint. The initial inflammatory factors that occur on a daily basis cause pain in the joints and the subsequent arrival of

Stems on the scene calms down the inflammation. Inflammation and the healing process doesn't actually create new cartilage so the body attempts the same process over and over again. The fact that the body continually attempts to repair these cartilage injuries is the reason that the body cycles through periods of inflammation leading to bad days, and the subsequent repair attempts, which lead to good days.

It is easy now to understand the general principle of harvesting Stems from your own body and injecting them into painful joints to try to decrease the inflammatory process. The fact is, Stems are anti-inflammatory cells and products that we have yet to fully understand. What we do understand very well from the literature and research is that the Stems are undeniably anti-inflammatory. We now have the ability to decrease our pain despite the fact that the cartilage will never be repaired to its original state. As far as I'm concerned, I would much rather use Stems in my joints than replace them with metal and plastic. Even if ultimately a joint has to be replaced, it makes much more sense to try to decrease inflammation around the joint for as long as we can to maintain our own anatomical structures before violating it will large incisions, saws, hammers, metal and plastic.

CHAPTER 6: STEMS

What are stems? How do they work? How do we keep them healthy?

The answer to these questions are the key to not only your health, but your very survival.

When I was finishing up my Applied Biology degree at Georgia Tech in 1988, the biology department was very small and housed in an upper floor of a peripheral building on campus. There weren't many students within this major, and most of them went on to go to medical school or become PHDs in other areas of science.

I had the opportunity to visit the campus of Georgia Tech in the last few years, and was shocked that there is now a massive building with many floors devoted just to bio-technology and biological sciences. In addition, there is another sector of campus that was devoted to nanotechnology which also dabbles in medical applications.

It became quite clear to me upon my visit to Georgia Tech, that times have changed significantly with the thoughts and hopes of wonder cures in the medical revolution based on treatment at the cellular level.

Stems (as I like to call them for short) are cells and their products that exist in the body. This includes not only humans, but also animals and the plant world. As we go through our initial growth in the embryonic stages, stems are the initial cells that are created at conception. They then begin to divide and create different structures of the body. In other words, stems are cells that have the ability to transform themselves into various forms and structures in the body, as well as the ability to heal defects and injuries to the body. As we also now know these stems have an anti-inflammatory effect comparable to medicines such as ibuprofen. Without stems we simply would not exist, or survive.

The health of our stems as we go through life is vital to help repair both external and internal injuries.

I give you the example of a child running down the street then tripping and falling and scraping both knees. Both knees will begin to bleed and then there's a process that takes place in the body that initiates platelets traveling to the scrapes on the knees to stop the bleeding. The platelets and the other factors that go to this site in the body for healing also have an inflammatory effect (yes they actually flare-up the injury site). That is why when someone falls or cuts themselves (or scrapes their knees) the wounds will look very inflamed, swollen and be very painful in the initial few days before the true scab or clotting begins to give way to stem repair of these sites.

The initial platelets and other healing factors including specific proteins in the body have a very aggressive effect on the injury site to ward off infection, stop bleeding and create a stable scab that walls off the inside of the body from external contamination. The next step in the process involves the stem cells being activated to make their way to this injured area and begin decreasing inflammation, repairing the site, and laying down new cells that will morphologically change into the injury site tissue.

In other words, if you injure your skin over your knee, the cells that will come to the knee tend to change into the type of skin that overlies the knee. Likewise, if you injure the skin or cartilage on the ear, the stems would eventually transform into the type of skin and tissue around the ear.

The mystery in medicine these days is how to make Stems work on internal disease in the body when the disease overwhelms the body's natural defenses. Research that is underway involves an attempt to find the cure for cancers, as well as chronic diseases such as multiple sclerosis, hepatitis, etc. In other words, there is an overwhelming and palpable effort among the scientists of today to use these stems to create a new medical revolution.

This revolution has now arrived. Just recently I was watching an NBA game on television and there were at least 3 athletes referenced who had undergone stem cell treatments for knees, shoulders and ankles. These were not second tier athletes, but rather top tier athletes and marquee names in the game of basketball.

Many of us have seen stories of athletes traveling to Germany or other countries to get their stem cell treatments and this has seemed very unattainable to most of us, until now. The technology and the ability now exists for anyone who is injured to consider the use of Stems for viable treatment for these injuries.

The FDA has been hot on the trail of the improper use of Stems. I personally am glad they've done this, given the fact that there have been so many false claims made during these early stages of bringing Stems to the general public. Multiple clinics have made false claims about creating new cartilage, new organs, and eradicating chronic disease long before any evidence existed that this could take place. It is a shame that we have to witness these charlatans try to go out and damage the reputation of the use of Stems for medical treatment.

What we currently know about Stems is that they do have an anti-inflammatory effect. This is enough to make me very excited about the future treatments of orthopedic injuries. The reality is that Stems cannot regrow cartilage inside the body, but the anti-inflammatory effect of Stems can make damaged cartilage be painless, or have less pain in the injured patient. I give you the example an elderly patients who I occasionally see in the office, saying that their knee just started hurting within the last 6 months. I then go and obtain an x-ray of the knee only to find that there has not been any cartilage in their knees for at least a decade, and there is nothing but bone on bone contact in the knee. I find myself asking the patient "how in the world have you not had any pain until a few months ago?" They often respond with statements such as "I have a good diet that includes nuts, berries, yogurt and other various anti-inflammatory foods." In addition, some people simply have very active stems that suppress inflammation without any difficulty. In other words, some individuals have the ability to quickly fight off inflammation because their stems are very healthy, active, and quick to react to any flare up in injured cartilage in the body. If only we were all so lucky.

If you are one of the individuals who do not have active healthy stems that quickly react to cartilage flare ups in the body, then you are probably experiencing pain, whether it be constant or occasional, due to the inflammation in the joints of your body. The traditional method of initially treating this pain is the use of ice, maintaining range of motion, maintaining flexibility and the occasional use of anti-inflammatory medicines such as ibuprofen. These methods have proven moderately successful and can certainly prolong the life of a healthy joint. When joints get significantly painful enough that these methods are not working, the standard traditional treatment is to get a "cortisone shot." This also has some good evidence to support its use and I personally use this method in clinic for occasional flare-ups for joints. The problem is that the patient can't come to the office every month and get a cortisone shot into a particular joint. The reason is because cortisone, although an anti-inflammatory also has an element of degrading the joint. In other words, to put it simply, although the cortisone shot might make you feel better its also damaging the very cartilage that you are trying to calm down or make feel better. Therefore, cortisone has very limited use on a long term repetitive basis.

The next step in treatment would consist of the use of gel shots or what has been termed Viscoelastic supplementation. These treatments include multiple injections over several weeks for a joint in order to increase the viscosity of the joint fluid (to make it glide better). Many patients do say that these injections give them good relief. However many patients indicate that they have no improvement whatsoever and have reported increased pain in the joints. I use these injections in the clinic as reasonable treatments for joints, particularly knees, that have become more chronically painful and have failed the more traditional treatments.

With regard to the use of PRP, (otherwise known as platelet rich plasma) this is obtained by drawing some blood from the patient, placing the blood in a centrifuge, and spinning the centrifuge to allow the PRP to rise to the top of the test tube. This material is then removed from the test tube and injected into the damaged joint of the patient. The idea of this treatment is to initiate a process similar to a new injury. The platelets and other clotting/healing factors initiate a repair in the joint that ultimately signals the stems to come to that site. I have noticed with patients with PRP injections that quite often they actually feel pain in the initial stages of the treatment although ultimately may receive some relief as the Stems make their way to the damaged joint. Therefore, the PRP injections do have the ultimate goal of decreasing inflammation although they use an initial inflammatory phase to make this happen.

Now we come to Stems. If you have been following the logic here, you have probably already asked the question, "If we're ultimately looking for stems to come in to decrease inflammation, why don't we just go and put Stems into the painful area to begin with?" If you have asked yourself this question you have identified the "holy grail" which creates billions of dollars in research and millions of hours of scientists working in laboratories around the world. The magic question is, "if we take the Stems and put them into a damaged area, how do we make those Stems transform into new cartilage, muscle, tendon, or blood cells?" The answer to this question is still elusive at this point in time in our medical history. However, there has been some encouraging progress in the treatment of leukemia and other blood diseases with use of embryonic stem cells.

Having identified the goal in medical treatment we now know that these Stems do have the ability to repair. Although we haven't figured out how to make them create new body parts yet, what we do know (and what the professional athletes are taking advantage of) is that these Stems have an anti-inflammatory effect that is undeniable.

If you will pay attention to the commentary during professional sports, such as basketball, football, soccer, track and field, and even golf, you will hear that certain athletes have gone for Stem treatments. The Stems that these athletes have used, have for the most part been their own Stems taken from their bodies. They are then prepared and re-injected into injured body parts for assistance in decreasing pain and attempts at healing.

You as the reader can now recognize why it is so critical to keep your stems healthy. They are literally the currency of your lifespan. If you keep your Stems healthy, they will fight for you in decreasing pain and healing injuries that occur externally and internally.

Getting back to the FDA, I must say that Stems are one example where the FDA has served an excellent role in quality control. The FDA has recently initiated policies to make it more difficult to take fat from the body and process it for re-injection. The purpose in doing this is to make sure that doctors and scientists recognize that fat has a vital role in protecting nerves, vessels, and support of other anatomic structures.

The FDA, at the time of me writing this book, in the early months of 2016, has not created stringent criteria for obtaining Stems from the iliac crest or pelvic bone, but certainly is keeping a close eye on clinics throughout the country, making sure that no false claims or inappropriate procedures are being performed. The patient needs to be informed about what Stems can and cannot do. This is a crucial step in the educational process of the public so they are aware of what is occurring within their own bodies. With the use of Stems there are risks. These risks need to be understood by the patient as well as the physician using them. The biggest risk initially is infection. Typically a patient is put in position on the procedure table and the skin sterilized. A needle is then placed down into the pelvic bone, and approximately 60cc (about a half of a coffee cup full of fluid) is then taken from the bone marrow. This fluid is then put in a centrifuge to spin the stems out of the solution. These stems are then prepared in a sterile environment and placed into a syringe and re-injected into a painful joint in the body. The infection risk also exists at the site of the injection. So in other words if stem treatment is being given there is a risk of infection at the area of the body where the Stems are taken from, and at the area of the body where they are placed (re-injected). The physician may choose to use antibiotic to prevent infection or rely on the sterilization of the skin alone to achieve this result. The bottom line is, that Stem treatment does have some risk.

The other risk that is present is to keep in mind that since Stems have the ability to transform into different types of tissue within the body, occasionally a Stem injection can be given into a joint and there can be some calcification (calcium deposits) created in these joints. This is why it is so important that Stems not be the initial treatment for every painful joint. Using stems in the treatment regimen should take place after more conservative treatments have been attempted.

Now that you have gone through the current philosophy, regiments, and goals of modern medicine with the use of Stems, I invite you to educate yourself further with some of the research that has been done in the last 10 years. There have been hundreds of publications and research papers in the last 10 years discussing the effective use of Stems, including what Stems can and can't do. A simple Google search for stem cell treatment, will provide you with more than enough information for review.

I welcome you into the world of stem cell treatment. Once you have educated yourself and are aware of the risk and benefits of Stems, you will be equipped, along with your physician, to make informed decisions as to whether you are a candidate for this revolutionary treatment.

CHAPTER 7: TRENDS IN MEDICINE

Going back about 40 years, you would have probably picked up a magazine in any waiting room and noticed doctors were supporting the use of cigarette smoking. By now we are all well aware of the fraud that was taking place by the tobacco companies. We're also aware that doctors were receiving payments to support the use of cigarettes.

It became quite clear in the subsequent years that cigarette smoking was perhaps the single worst activity that an individual could do, causing cancers, decreased function of vital organs and ultimately, early death. This is not even to mention the quality of life that was stolen from individuals by the false claims from tobacco companies along with physicians support.

I remember when I started my private practice in 1997, that when I went around to visit other physicians to get referrals for my practice, there were at least 3 physicians offices that I walked in that the physicians themselves were smoking and had ashtrays throughout their office. It wasn't long prior to this that there were actually smoking areas for the physicians and patients in the hospitals with ashtrays strewn about the hospitals. It was not unheard of to walk into a physicians office to see them smash their cigarette in an ashtray before walking into an exam room to take care of the medical needs of a patient making recommendations regarding a healthy lifestyle.

It's safe to say that with regard to cigarette smoking and diet we have come a long way in the last 60 years. Not so long ago MRI scans did not exist. An MRI scan is a magnetic imaging technique to take pictures of the inside of the body. It has become so routine now in the field of medicine to obtain an MRI that it is hard to imagine a time where they did not exist. Nearly every patient who presents to an orthopedic office with an ailment that has failed conservative management will end up with an MRI scan of that particular joint or body part. There is no radiation and it only uses magnets.

I remember very well when the initial MRI scans became available. All physicians alike wondered what ailments we had missed in the past by not using the MRI scan as a screening tool for patients.

I also remember a certain time in my training in the early 1990s when certain older physicians would say MRI scans were "over doing it" or "I don't need an MRI I can tell by just examining the patient." The concept of a physical exam being able to provide all the answers proved to be incredibly false as there are many injuries and ailments that cannot be detected unless an MRI scan is performed.

With regard to mammograms this is also a phenomenon in medicine that has provided the wonderful ability to pre-screen for breast cancers and tumors long before they are detectable by physician examination.

When it comes to the general notion of using stems for medical treatment, clearly there is still a lot of work to be done. It is my opinion that the education of the public regarding stems is key in its acceptance for treatments of ailments in our society. The simple fact is we possess within our bodies the tremendous potential to heal ourselves, although sometimes there are some barriers to the stems reaching the injury site.

Take for example an average joint such as a knee, shoulder, or hip. As a mature adult the cartilage lining of those joints simply does not have very good blood supply. Therefore, since there is not a good blood supply there is no way for the stems to appropriately reach the inner aspect of the joint to fight off inflammation and attempt cartilage repair and maintenance. If one is aware of this fact, it is clear to see that obtaining stems from one area of the body and preparing them for injection into another area of the body that does not have good blood supply, such as a joint makes perfectly good sense. Certainly there is a tremendous amount of research that already supports the use of stems for this purpose. However, much research is yet to be done regarding the mechanism of actions helping not only decrease inflammation but cure diseases and increase the amount of repair that can be done by stems within the patient's body.

The oath that medical students take when they become physicians on their final day of medical school is the Hippocratic Oath. Within this oath is the concept of "do no harm." There could be no greater guidance in medicine today than this simple statement. This applies to stems as it does to any other medical treatment that exists. I for one am following the current research closely and participating in my own clinical research in our clinic. I am determined to make sure that each and every patient that enters my office understands what Stems are, how they work, and what the risk and benefits are to their use. The patient needs to understand that there are more conservative methods that may work for them and these should be tried before embarking on Stem treatments. However, when conservative treatment has failed and the only remaining steps are joint replacement or severe disability with use of crutches or canes, Stems have come of age to help fill this gap and provide decreased pain in these joints.

If you are reading this book and wondering if you are a candidate for Stem treatments for painful joints, keep a few key things in mind. First of all it's important to remember that there are diets that are anti-inflammatory. The very foods you eat can help decrease painful joints along with supplements including glucosamine/chondroitin-sulfate taken on a daily basis.

Additionally you should make sure that you are maintaining a healthy lifestyle with no smoking, moderation in alcohol consumption, and a balanced diet. Stretching and light conditioning exercises are also important in maintaining joint health.

Once a joint begins to hurt with any kind of inflammatory process, whether it is arthritis, or a flare up from repetitive use, certain principles have applied in the past and still apply today. This includes the judicious use of ice and anti-inflammatory's such as ibuprofen, as well as compression and elevation for acute flare-ups. If you have tried all of these traditional methods and there is still pain then it is time to start discussing with your physician the role of Stems. Like any injection or procedure, Stems have risks, but using cortisone on a repetitive basis has a risk of joint destruction and gel shots have a shared risk of infection as well.

Anyone who is considering Stems for their painful joints should definitely check their family history to make sure that there is no history of rheumatoid arthritis or other inflammatory diseases. It would certainly be good to be evaluated by an internal medicine doctor to make sure none of these are the primary underlying sources of joint pain. Once these sources of inflammation have been ruled out and more conservative methods of painful joint treatment have been exhausted, Stems start to become a more viable option and a discussion with your physician regarding Stems can then ensue.

As you the reader embark on educating yourself about Stems and considering them for yourself, I welcome you to the new world of medicine and the advantages of Stem treatments in preventing further pain and increasing healthy active lifestyles. Stem treatments will become more actively pursued by physicians and the general public as time passes and advances will be made, not only in understanding the use of Stems but also in the clinical use of Stems for us all. I welcome you to this new world of modern medicine that has existed within us all along.

CHAPTER 8: MEDITATION

It's hard to imagine sitting and thinking of nothing. The reality is, that is exactly what our Stems need each day. Research has shown us that time spent in quiet reflection without disturbances from the world around us supports the immune system and subsequently the health of Stems. The ability to control blood pressure, keep our daily stress to a manageable level and take on problems that appear bigger than ourselves are all enhanced by this short time each day of thinking of nothing.

Some individuals may prefer to hum or direct their thoughts toward a higher being. These are some of the methods of meditation and without question support an ongoing healthy lifestyle.

Surveying religious and non-religious orders across the world reveals one thing that is a common thread throughout. That one thing is the time that each of these organizations commit to some sort of prayer, meditation, or quiet thought. There must be something to this given how ubiquitous it is throughout the world. In fact, it is clearly supported by medical research showing the health benefits of such an activity.

It's easy to get caught up in our lives of working, taking care of children and meeting financial goals and needs. It's equally important for us to recognize that the efforts to achieve these goals and perform these activities take a toll on our Stems. The ability to fight off infection, maintain healthy bone and muscle and have an overall upbeat view of our lives depends on not only physical health but mental health as well. Both physical and mental health, depend on quiet introspection each day.

I've discussed this with people in various religions over the years including the practitioners of transcendental meditation. There is no doubt if you find yourself going an entire week without taking 20 minutes per day to sit down by yourself in quiet without the distractions of the world around, it will ultimately lead to poor health and early demise.

To a lot of people it almost seems silly to take this time to themselves and some may even think it is selfish. The reality is it is not selfish at all. Without taking these periods of time for meditation, prayer, or deep introspection, we are unable to better serve those around us. Quite often it's hard to get away from the distractions of the day including cell phones, televisions, jobs, and children. We must make it known to those around us that we are going to dedicate some time to this practice of introspection so everyone around us will respect that time alone.

I challenge you to develop a pattern of meditation, prayer, or deep introspection that occurs every day for a minimum of 20 minutes. I'm confident you will find if you truly clear your mind for 20 minutes and block out the world around, you will see a dramatic improvement of your outlook on life, health, and well being after 6 weeks. In fact, I anticipate that after 6 weeks it will be such a habit forming practice for you that it will be hard not to have this time to yourself.

With regard to the health of your Stems, it is essential to dedicate yourself to this quiet time on a daily basis so they can recharge and be ready to fight the next battle.

CHAPTER 9: SLEEP

In 1992 when I started my surgical internship and residency in Atlanta I wasn't aware that full nights of sleep were pretty much over. When I was in my surgical residency in the 1990's it was prior to some of the laws that have now been passed, limiting the number of hours interns and residents can work in a hospital per week.

The surgical program in which I was involved, required frequent 36 hour shifts and every few weeks required 72 hour shifts. I know this sounds unbelievable but it is actually true. Frequently I would arrive at work on Friday mornings at the Georgia Baptist Medical Center and be working or on call until Monday evening. I was able to go and rest in a "call room." It usually consisted of a small bed and a single locker but actually served to provide little rest at all. In those days I carried a beeper and there was a phone present in the call room. It was not uncommon to have the beeper go off every one to two hours for the entire 72 hour shift and have to make multiple trips back and forth to the emergency room, hospital ward, and operating room every night. There were some Monday afternoons when I would leave the hospital after 72 straight hours and I would have forgotten what the outside looked like and what it felt like to feel the sunshine. When I look back now I'm not quite sure how I, or others, survived with this relentless beat down of work and lack of sleep for five years. I can't help but wonder why it took so long for the surgical residency programs to come to the realization that this was an extremely unhealthy lifestyle. It has only been in recent years that new rules have limited the amount of hours that medical residents can work in a hospital. I can only assume that it was the idea from the older physicians that said "well we did it, so you have to do it." Fortunately, logic won in the long run and the new rules in place allow medical residents and interns to work hard but also have time to get appropriate rest and personal time.

It wasn't until a few years after I finished my residency that I was able to teach myself how to sleep well at night. During my first few years in private practice I was still in the habit of only getting about four uninterrupted hours of sleep per night and found myself awake many times at 4 and 5 in the morning with the inability to get back to sleep.

In todays world with the many distractions and life stressors that come at us everyday it is equally important for every individual to get an appropriate amount of sleep to allow the body to recover. Needless to say our Stems derive their health from not only the nutrition that feeds them, but also the amount of rest they obtain. Giving Stems time to recover and reboot for the next assault is essential in maintaining the health of the body.

These days there are multiple medications available to get a good night sleep, however, there are some medications prescribed by physicians that may help us get sleep but don't allow us to go through the proper sleep cycles to give our bodies the appropriate rest needed. It is important to discuss with your physician not only which medication may help you rest but also what side effects and anticipated sleep patterns you can expect from that particular medicine.

An example of a medicine that is taken frequently today is Ambien. Great success has been reported with the use of this medication but if this medication is used, it must be used at the appropriate time with the individual being able to dedicate a significant amount of time to rest and recovery. Every individual is certainly different and it requires a conversation with your physician to determine what is a safe dosage and frequency of use for this medication.

Ideally it would be best to never take medication so other methods of trying to achieve a good night sleep should certainly be tried as well. Some of these methods are very simple such as a brisk walk in the evening after dinner, which has been proven to not only help individuals stay conditioned but also provides great psychological advantages. Making sure that we eat healthy, avoiding certain food and drinks that stimulate the body in the evenings is critical for a good night sleep. Whether you like it or not, symphony or new age music has been shown to help promote an earlier and longer night of sleep.

There are many natural products on the market as well that provide a good night sleep. There is a lot of trial and error involved in the use of medications- whether they be holistic or physician prescribed, so I encourage you to be skeptical of every medication you are prescribed until you find the one that works best for you. Don't let marketing campaigns of Wall-street traded companies convince you of what works best for sleep, make the decision about what works for best for you and resist the latest fad.

I encourage you to attempt more natural methods prior to embarking on a medication regimen that may become habit-forming and difficult to break as the years pass.

There are experts available these days that can provide sleep studies for an individual who has difficulty sleeping. A sleep study may require you to spend the night with monitoring to assess the patterns of sleep that you experience. It sounds like it may be a little bit over the top to go through this type of testing for every individual, however if you think about it, a single night testing that could help you get good sleep for the rest of your life is worth the cost.

As I think back to those times in the hospital when I was putting in the long hours and shifts, I remember walking around the halls passing other doctors while we blankly stared at each other. Now that I think of it, we must have looked like a bunch of zombies walking around the hospital. I find that it's not just medical residents that experience these unhealthy sleep patterns, but many of us find ourselves awake in the middle of the night worrying about the concerns of the day including financial, family, and work stressors. We can learn a lot from individuals in other cultures who dedicate the time to not only get a good night sleep but also rest in the middle of the day. It is probably unrealistic to expect us in the United States to take two hour lunches and get 8-9 hours sleep every night, but it's a goal that's worth the effort.

CHAPTER 10: GOING ON TILT

In the last decade we witnessed the rise of Texas hold'em as the premier and sexy way to play poker. It started with a win by Chris Moneymaker seen the world over as he defeated a field of many thousands of individuals to win the title.

In the subsequent years it became a common phrase to say "going on tilt." This term basically means things start to go bad at the poker table by either losing a hand that you thought you were going to win or not getting any playable cards and watching your money dwindle away. What follows is a series of unwise decisions about how to play the hand you are dealt and eventually the loss of all your money. This same principle applies to managing our own health. Think about it. We can be going along fine with exercise and diet and then some major life event occurs such as divorce, death of a loved one, or losing a job and all the sudden our health takes a serious hit. It's very common when experiencing these life situations to resort to comfort foods that are not very good for us and to abandon exercise for more escapist activities such as drinking and smoking.

It is in these tough times in life when we should actually be concentrating more on healthy habits and lifestyles. Most of the time there is a light at the end of the tunnel. If we can manage to get through the tunnel of life's stresses by maintaining our health and fitness and keeping our Stems ready to react and heal internal and external injuries, we'll find that we come out the other side ready to take on the new world of circumstances we face. I'm sure we all know individuals who we thought had everything going for them and then all of the sudden some tragedy or adverse event occurred in their life that lead to a major decline and sometimes even demise that we would have never expected.

Going back to the poker reference this would be termed "going on tilt" with regard to our health. It is one of the most dangerous activities to participate in, and once it starts it is very difficult to stop. It becomes very important for us as individuals to maintain social networking throughout life including friends and family, so that when we are unable to stop the slide in health and well being ourselves, we are close enough with friends and family that they can reach out with a helping hand. We must be open with our friends and family so they feel open enough with us to step in and give a guiding word or action in times of need.

It's almost innate within us to want to help others we see going downhill fast and we want others to help us when we are experiencing a downturn.

If we can keep our Stems healthy during these trying times in life we will be less susceptible to cancers, emotional and psychological breakdowns, and other ailments that effect us such as diabetes and heart disease. It seems so simple when we sit and read a book, however, when these events are actually happening to us, it seems nearly impossible to pull ourselves out and maintain the discipline of a healthy lifestyle.

The reason I included this section in this book was to point out the importance of maintaining social networks around us with friends and family who are in the loop and ready to step in to keep us on the straight and narrow with regard to health and fitness.

In addition to my Beverly Hills practice, I have spent many years now going to Bakersfield to run a clinic twice a month. I usually spend the night in a local hotel just off the highway in the center of town. Every morning I wake up, go to the gym, shower and then partake in the wonderful breakfast buffet that is available to guests of the hotel. I cant help but notice almost every time I go to the breakfast buffet on Thursday mornings there is a group of older women, most of them in their 70s or 80s, that meet for an obvious planned social gathering. Every week it's the same women that are smiling, happy, and thoroughly engaged in conversation with good friends. I use this as an example to myself to ensure that I maintain healthy relationships and friendships as time passes. It becomes easy to want to become reclusive, and hideaway with our problems when in fact the exact opposite should occur. Taking the initiative to maintain supportive relationships and scheduled social gatherings is just as healthy as going to the gym or avoiding smoking. Our Stems respond to all kinds of stimuli, not only from diet and exercise but also from laughter, joy, and a lack of depression and anxiety. Planned social gatherings such as what I witness in Bakersfield hold the keys to our psychological health and adds another piece of the puzzle in maintaining the effectiveness of our Stems.

CHAPTER 11: RHYTHM OF HEALTH

John Grisham is by far my favorite writer. Born in Arkansas he then went on to attend multiple Universities and create a dynasty of legal and non-legal thrillers.

I had the opportunity to listen to John Grisham speak at a local University in Cleveland, Mississippi several years ago. I was fascinated by the stories he told and the books he had written.

Grisham was very quiet and pensive not only while giving his lecture but in the pre- and post-lecture social gathering with those around him. I've always enjoyed his writing but at that time I started enjoying the man's outlook and perspective on the world.

I learned a very valuable lesson from him. That lesson is the importance of working, even if you don't need to financially, and continuing that work on a regimented schedule.

Grisham discussed how he was a baseball fan and how he had participated in not only little league baseball but also enjoyed watching professional baseball as an adult and recounted tales of listening to the St. Louis Cardinals play when he was a boy. Grisham indicated that during baseball season it was time to concentrate on baseball and when the World Series was over it was time to write a new book. He seemed to imply that this was his yearly schedule. I got the impression that after the World Series every year he sat down to write a new book and tried to complete it before spring training. I don't know the man, but this is what he seemed to suggest in his lectures. Of course I wondered why would a successful writer such as this who is clearly financially stable, put himself on a regimented program and deadline of writing a new novel every year between the end of the World Series and spring training? During the past few years it has become clear to me that work and social interactions at work are key in maintaining the health of your Stems. This social interaction is clearly not only a support in our personal lives, but also our work lives. It would seem that deadlines and regimented work schedules are healthy. In fact, research shows us this. It is quite clear that those individuals that maintain reasonable work schedules and regimented deadlines live longer happier lives with less psychological problems than those who work intermittent schedules or those who do not work at all.

I suppose it must be some kind of rhythm that our bodies get into that allows us to gather energy for work and then schedule downtimes when the work is complete. This is in contrast to someone who is not working or remaining active. That persons schedule becomes guesswork for the body with no form or fashion. The body does not have a deadline to strive for therefore it does not know when it can rest.

Little did I know when I went to hear Grisham talk, I would not just be learning about the ideas that drove some of his incredibly captivating novels, but more importantly I would learn how a successful individual maintains health and happiness in their everyday life.

CHAPTER 12: POOPOLOGY

My wife affectionately refers to me as a poopologist.

She typically has to remind me prior to any social gatherings or cocktail parties that it would probably be a good idea if I tried to refrain from asking people about their bowel functions. Not that I would randomly bring this subject up, but if someone starts to ask me about a physical ailment I almost always will ask how their bowels are functioning.

I find it hard not to do so when people start to ask me about their orthopedic problems such as joint pains, muscle aches, and limitation of function. Based on my training in medical school and residency, I closely associate food intake and excretion with quality of life and health of our Stems.

Stems rely not only on the food we eat but also on the ability of our body to excrete toxins that are detrimental to their health.

Most of us aren't aware but as we digest our foods and rid our bodies of the waste it is very easy for much of this waste to get trapped in our bowels and linger for weeks and even months. Trapped bowel contents sit in the small corners of our bowels and continually give off toxins to the blood supply that flows through the liver and to the remainder of our body.

It's easy to forget this fact because even if you are having normal bowel movements everyday, it is still quite often that there are remaining bowel contents that remain trapped.

It's easy to think of our digestive system as a simple smooth tube that runs from our mouth to our stomach then leading to the exit far below. The reality is once the food leaves our stomach for processing, it follows a torturous route. Not only do our bowels have many twists and turns but there are many bulges of the bowels along the way. If the ability to absorb the proper nutrients in our digestive tract is not functioning normally we leave many of the toxic contents of our bowels behind, trapped in these bulges and poisoning our system.

There are common ways to help cleanse our bowels including herbals, prescription medications, and enemas. I highly recommend that each individual invest the time and money into visiting at least once in their adult life a nutrition and digestive tract expert. Understanding the food we eat and how it is processed is essential to making good diet decisions. The food that passes through our system nourishes our Stems and ultimately determines our everyday energy and ability to fight inflammation and infection.

Quite often we eat what we think is a healthy anti-inflammatory diet as well as avoid smoking and excessive alcohol use, yet our bowels still might not be working normally. The reality is our bowels are very responsive to emotional life stressors.

An extremely common condition in our society is IBS or Irritable Bowel Syndrome. IBS is a condition in which a patient may experience bloating, stomach pain, abnormal bowel movements, and ultimately suffer from poor nutrition, fatigue and disease even though that patient may be eating correctly. IBS conditions are quite often genetic, being passed down through family trees, but also have a significant emotional component related to how we handle our daily life stressors. It is important to maintain the health of our bowels by limiting life stressors that contribute to the emotional component of this disease. Controlling the environment around us to keep our emotional stressors to a minimum will keep our Stems healthy, rested, and ready for action.

It is important to not only rest the body but also the mind. The ability to compartmentalize daily problems is of the utmost importance in order to avoid a constant assault on our Stems of stressors that result in high blood pressure, diabetes, and IBS.

Many of us don't think about it much, but the health of our thyroid and adrenal glands is essential in fueling the engine that keeps us on the move everyday. Stems will quickly respond to injuries if the hormone and electrolyte balance in our bodies is in synch.

Exercise is intimately involved in the processing of the foods we eat and fluids we drink. Exercise however, can be detrimental if we do too high of intensity for prolonged periods of time. The simple fact is that if we don't regulate the degree of exercise that we perform it is easy to exhaust our Stems and essentially wear out our adrenals. The adrenal glands sit just above our kidneys and the substances they secrete control our metabolism.

I give you an example of an individual that goes to the gym everyday and performs one hour of intense aerobic activity. This individual is certainly giving themselves many benefits but if the body does not have a chance to rest and there are not periods of low intensity alternating with high intensity exercise, the adrenal glands can very easily get burned out and compensate with a hyperactive bowel and a general feeling of fatigue and depression.

Stems rely on us keeping the toxins away from them. The adrenal glands and the thyroid are regulators of our bodies not becoming over exerted or too fatigued. Maintaining a proper mineral balance through healthy diet along with anti-inflammatory foods can be the difference in making it through a day without having the fatigue that keeps us from enjoying what we are doing with family and friends, as well as performing work.

When a patient comes to my office and I have an opportunity to speak with him or her about any chronic joint pain or muscle fatigue the conversation always turns to nutrition. It is probably more important for an individual to be aware of what is a proper diet, including vitamin and mineral supplementation, than any other aspect regarding the health of our Stems. Understanding how the body moves and how to protect it from injury is important from an orthopedic standpoint, but how the body is fueled and knowing what foods keep it running smoothly without getting overheated is equally important.

Once again I can't over-emphasize how important it is to at least once during your adult life, sit down with a trained nutritionist and understand how food affects your bodily functions. In most cases its easy for us to think we have full knowledge of this by watching TV shows or from high school biology class, but the fact is that there are many aspects of nutrition, bowel function, and the maintenance of our metabolism that are simply not taught or easily learned without sitting down with an appropriate expert.

As you embark on your self-education in the field of poopology I encourage you to keep a written log of the foods you eat and your pattern of bowel movements. You will be shocked at what this will reveal to you about how your food is processed and how it directly relates to not only your energy levels but also your pain levels with any chronic orthopedic conditions or diseases.

No discussion about the health of the digestive system would be complete without addressing oral health. You may not realize it but our Stems are hard at work repairing problems in the mouth including gingivitis, receding gum lines, and chronic infections.

A routine of brushing, flossing, and rinsing with appropriate mouthwash to externally fight infection is essential in preserving the energy of Stems for fights in other locations that we can not as easily address.

One of my friends who is a dental hygienist has commented to me on several occasions that it is surprising to her that a patient will come to her office and have the appearance of being a well educated professional, yet when they open their mouth for a teeth cleaning they have plaque build up, receding gum lines and infections. She indicates that there seems to be an epidemic of individuals that become more advanced in their careers but they will disregard flossing and oral health and defer to a dental hygienist to clean their mouths every 3 months. This is the worst possible scenario when someone is actually educated about taking care of their mouth and chooses to dump the responsibility on someone else when a nightly routine of brushing, flossing and rinsing appropriately is essential to fighting off the constant assault on our teeth and gums by bacteria. Once again it would be much easier to do these routines on our own and let our Stems rest to fight another day.

CHAPTER 13: FAT TO THE RESCUE

I hope your sitting down for this next part. That fat around your waist and thighs is not only a source of Stems but may very well save your life someday. In fact, your fat may have already saved your life and you don't even know how or when.

One of the most recent treatments brought to market over the last year is the use of fat to treat painful joints. The process involves you, as a patient, undergoing a liposuction procedure to remove fat from your body (usually from the waist or thighs). This fat is then rinsed gently with sterile fluid to cleanse the fat and prepare it for the next stage of treatment. The same fat that was removed from your body only minutes before is then injected into your painful joints to relieve pain. As unbelievable as it sounds the fat in your own body has already deployed Stems to areas of injury and disease and solved the problem without you even knowing that it occurred.

The Liposuction procedure that I am referring to can be done safely and without much discomfort under local anesthesia. If there is a joint in your body, such as a knee or hip, that is painful or arthritic and it is well worth your time to look into using your own fat to make you feel better.

In the past ten years there have been many clinics that have used the liposuction technique to obtain fat and then dissolve the fat with some materials that destroyed the internal make-up of the fat. The resulting dissolved fat would then be injected into a patient's vein. The idea was that this infusion into the body would decrease pain and make the patient feel better, particularly if there were any inflammatory conditions in the body such as rheumatoid arthritis or Lupus. The problem with this method was that the FDA did not approve the procedure due to the fact that the fat was broken down from it's original form and function to perform the injection. The newer technique of using sterile saline (a clear fluid similar to the makeup of the fluid in our own bodies) to minimally manipulate and cleanse the fat has recently garnered support from the FDA.

The concept of using the fat from your body to treat your pain is now a reality. Further uses of fat for treatment of other diseases are being actively researched and my opinion is we are only in the beginning stages of this amazing discovery.

CHAPTER 14: THE REVOLUTION HAS ARRIVED

Stems are powerhouse cells and products that exist in our bodies. They exist in a lot of areas of our body, but they are in retrievable concentrations in bone marrow and fat. Bone marrow is the inner aspect of the bone that is soft and has a good blood supply that is rich in nutrients. Fat is existent throughout our bodies but certain locations are more easily accessible, such as the abdomen and thighs.

Stems have an amazing ability to transform themselves into multiple types of tissues and structures in our bodies. They are essentially the final building block and repair mechanism for injuries that occur both to the inside and outside of our bodies.

A good example would be a child who is running and falls down and scrapes both knees and both hands with a lot of bleeding in these areas. The body will immediately send platelets and other reactors to the site to stop the bleeding and start the inflammatory process with a scab. The Stems are then triggered to make their way to these injured knees and hands to begin the process of repairing the skin and laying down new skin underneath to restore the original anatomy. This extraordinary process that takes place within us is essentially an internal hospital that creates and provides all of the tools to heal ourselves from injury. We take this phenomenon for granted every day because we are so used to being able to heal our own wounds we forget about the magic happening inside.

Think of the very process of conception in human beings, or in any mammal for that matter. There is a small sperm cell that joins with a small egg cell, and these two cells have all the genetic information and power to create another living being. This process of conception and growth is an example of how powerful certain cells in our body are to create new life, as well as heal injured tissue.

Without the existence of Stems in our bodies we would not survive very long. The Stems have a roving eye, always ready to quickly respond to injury and waiting their turn to perform the final healing steps in a process that has taken billions of years to develop.

Without going into all the science of the multiple proteins and enzymes involved, (which I'm sure we have all heard multiple times in biology class since grade school) I'd like to direct your attention to the extraordinary process that allows us to breathe and survive the harsh environment around us everyday. Our Stems are constantly at work repairing skin damage not only from abrasions and cuts, but also from sun exposure, heat, and cold. Now that you understand the process of how Stems come in to perform the final stages of healing it is easy to understand how any assault to these Stems including tobacco use, excessive alcohol use, excessive sun damage, and fatigue can have a deleterious effect on our bodies ability to heal itself. In fact most diseases are attributed to a breakdown in the repair process. These injuries may be traumatic such as falling down, or long-term injuries such as cancer, leukemia's, etc. If the Stems lose their ability to respond and repair we are left with wounds that are in a persistent and chronic state of attempted repair, leaving our body defenseless against bacteria and viruses. There is one area in our body that is particularly susceptible to chronic inflammation and that is the joints in our body. The cartilage that lines our joints does not have very good blood supply. The cartilage relies not only on the blood supply that comes in from arteries but also relies on the health of the joint fluid itself for nourishment. Joint fluid not only provides lubrication but also nutrients to the inner portion of the cartilage. If someone develops injury to the cartilage from some traumatic event or overuse, that cartilage breakdown not only decreases the smoothness of the joint but contributes to a decrease in nutrition to the remainder of the cartilage and therefor a snowball effect occurs. If the cartilage receives less joint fluid nourishment, it becomes more susceptible to a degenerative process to which Stems cannot react because they have no way to reach this final destination in our joints.

The above situation is exactly why there has been such a fevered pitch in the development of Stem technology. The ability to deliver Stems to damaged joints as well as using them to restore youthful qualities is the Holy Grail of medicine. The revolution that is now upon us involves the use of Stems in a way that nobody in the history of man has ever harnessed. Hundreds of research articles published over the last decade reveal that the anti-inflammatory effects of Stems are undeniable. The discovery of the use of Stems for our health and will eclipse the computer revolution as the most dramatic change in our society.

The current concept in the use of Stems to decrease joint pain is to go and take them from the body, prepare them outside of the body in high concentrations, and then re-inject them into joints to decrease inflammation and pain. It is important to understand that we are not reliably growing new cartilage with the Stems yet but we are decreasing pain and inflammation, which in turn increases function. There is also evidence now that points to the fact that Stems have the ability to force the body to create more blood vessels in areas where oxygen is lacking. For example, since a joint has very few blood vessels inside, injecting stems into a joint can increase the blood flow to that joint and therefore allow the body to get more anti-inflammatory factors to the joint on it's own in the future. As you can imagine, harnessing this power of Stems has great potential for the treatment of heart and lung disease.

The explanation that now presents itself to us through current research is that the fluctuating states of inflammation around damaged cartilage is what gives us our "good days" and our "bad days". This is further evidence that the pain we experience in joints is not necessarily the degeneration itself but rather the inflammatory process that takes place in an attempt to heal the damaged cartilage. Essentially what we are experiencing is waves of attempts at healing the cartilage with an initial inflammatory response followed by an attempt by Stems to decrease inflammation and heal. However, the Stems do not have as much ability to repair the cartilage because they are not reaching the cartilage in high enough concentrations over long enough periods of time.

The above principle is important to remember when we discuss obtaining Stems from one area of the body where they exist in high concentrations, then injecting them into joints where they do not have the ability to gather in high concentrations.

I am certain we ultimately will have the ability to not only decrease inflammation around damaged joints, but also manipulate Stems to restore and heal the original cartilage. Until we reach this milestone with the use of Stems the proper use of them for decreasing the inflammatory processes is going to rule the day in orthopedic offices around the world.

Welcome to the revolution my friends.